The Complete Whole30 Cookbook:

100 delicious recipes for your whole30 program

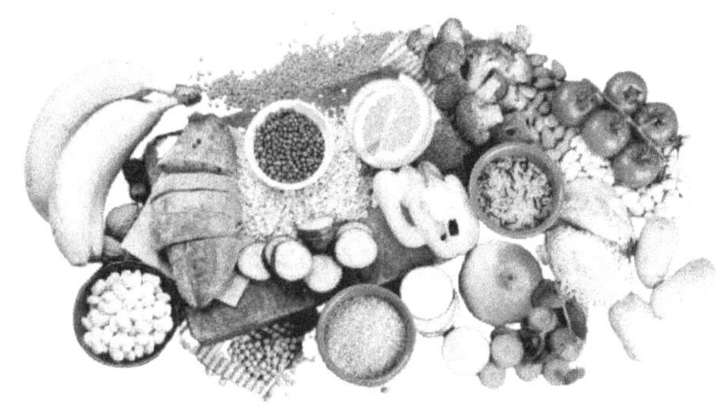

William Forge

Table Of Content

Introduction

Phil and Mitchell were two pals who had been suffering with their weight for years. They had tried several diets and fitness routines, but nothing seemed to work. Ultimately, they decided to attempt the Whole30 regimen.

At first, it was tough to make the move. They had to give up their favorite dishes and learn new recipes. Yet they were determined to continue with it, and soon they started to notice effects. The weight fell off, their energy levels soared, and they felt better than ever.

They also saw other good improvements in their lives. When they ate better, they began to have more energy to dedicate towards their occupations and pastimes. Their connections with friends and family improved, too, since they were more focused on their health and not on bad behaviors.

Phil and Mitchell persevered with the Whole30 regimen for 30 days, and towards the end of it, they felt like new people. They had both dropped weight, felt better, and were more inspired to continue on their objectives.

They chose to keep the program continuing and now, many months later, they're still following the Whole30 principles. They've both changed their lives tremendously, and they're appreciative for the improvement the program has made in their lives.

The Whole30 program is a 30-day nutritional reset meant to help individuals discover and resolve bad eating behaviors and build better habits with lasting results. The approach emphasizes avoiding particular food categories, such as dairy, grains, legumes, and alcohol while promoting the intake of full, unprocessed foods. The Whole30 program is aimed to help individuals build a better connection with food and their bodies. It stresses mindful eating, encourages individuals to listen to their bodies needs, and helps them make educated decisions about their nutrition so that people may improve their health, eliminate cravings, and establish a better lifestyle.

The suggested food plan for a whole30 regimen

The Whole30 regimen is a 30-day elimination diet that focuses on entire, unadulterated foods. It is meant to help reset your body by eliminating potentially inflammatory and harmful foods, while simultaneously providing you with satisfying, nutrient-dense meals.

The suggested meal plan for a Whole30 program comprises three meals and one snack each day. Each meal should contain a protein source, a healthy fat, and a vegetable or fruit. This is an example of a daily food plan:

Breakfast: Scrambled eggs with spinach, avocado, and tomatoes

Snack: Apple slices with almond butter

Lunch: Grilled salmon with roasted sweet potatoes and sautéed Brussels sprouts

Dinner: Grilled chicken with roasted asparagus and zucchini

The Whole30 program also supports nutrient-dense meals such as nuts, seeds, and healthy oils like olive or avocado oil. It also recommends lots of water and modest doses of coffee. Also, it's crucial to avoid added sugars, artificial sweeteners, and processed meals.

By following this meal plan, you may have wholesome meals that give your body the nutrition it needs to perform effectively. It may also help you reset your body and build healthy habits that will stay beyond the 30-day program.

Whole30 program breakfast recipes

Avocado Egg Cups:
Ingredients: 2 avocados, 4 eggs, 1/2 teaspoon sea salt, 1/4 teaspoon freshly ground black pepper
Instructions: Preheat oven to 350°F. Cut avocados in half, remove the pit and scoop out a bit of the flesh to create a large enough space for the egg. Crack one egg into each avocado half. Sprinkle with salt and pepper. Bake in preheated oven for 20 minutes.
Prep Time: 10 minutes

Zucchini Hash Browns:
Ingredients: 2 zucchini, 1 tablespoon olive oil, 2 cloves garlic, minced, 1/2 teaspoon sea salt
Instructions: Grate zucchini and place in a colander. Allow to sit for 10 minutes to drain off excess water. Heat a large skillet over

medium heat. Add olive oil and garlic and cook for 1 minute. Add grated zucchini and salt and cook for 10 minutes, stirring occasionally.
Prep Time: 15 minutes

Bacon and Egg Breakfast Burrito:
Ingredients: 4 slices bacon, 4 eggs, 1/4 cup chopped onion, 1/2 teaspoon sea salt, 1/4 teaspoon freshly ground black pepper, 4 whole-grain tortillas
Instructions: Preheat a large skillet over medium heat. Add bacon slices and cook for 5 minutes, flipping once. Remove bacon and set aside. In the same skillet, add eggs, onion, salt, and pepper. Cook for 5 minutes, stirring occasionally. Place each bacon slice and egg mixture in a tortilla and roll up.
Prep Time: 10 minutes

 Sweet Potato Breakfast Bowl:
Ingredients: 2 sweet potatoes, 1 tablespoon olive oil, 1/2 teaspoon sea salt, 1/4 teaspoon freshly ground black pepper, 1/4 cup

unsweetened almond milk, 1/4 cup almonds, 1/4 cup blueberries, 1/4 cup chopped fresh parsley

Instructions: Preheat oven to 400°F. Cut sweet potatoes into cubes and place on a baking sheet. Drizzle with olive oil, salt, and pepper. Roast for 30 minutes, stirring occasionally. Place cooked sweet potatoes in a bowl and pour almond milk over top. Top with almonds, blueberries, and parsley.

Prep Time: 10 minutes

<u>Turkey Sausage and Spinach Frittata:</u>

Ingredients: 4 eggs, 2 tablespoons milk, 1/2 teaspoon sea salt, 1/4 teaspoon freshly ground black pepper, 2 tablespoons olive oil, 1/2 cup chopped onion, 1/2 cup chopped red bell pepper, 1/2 cup chopped turkey sausage, 1/2 cup spinach

Instructions: Preheat oven to 350°F. In a bowl, whisk together eggs, milk, salt, and pepper. Heat a large oven-safe skillet over medium heat. Add olive oil, onion, bell pepper, turkey sausage, and spinach and

cook for 5 minutes, stirring occasionally. Pour egg mixture over the vegetables and cook for 5 minutes. Place skillet in preheated oven and bake for 15 minutes.
Prep Time: 10 minutes

Coconut Date Breakfast Bars:
Ingredients: 1 cup pitted dates, 1/2 cup unsweetened shredded coconut, 1/2 cup almond butter, 1/4 cup coconut oil, 1 teaspoon ground cinnamon
Instructions: Preheat oven to 350°F. Line a baking dish with parchment paper. In a food processor, combine dates, coconut, almond butter, coconut oil, and cinnamon. Process until a thick, dough-like consistency is formed. Transfer dough to prepared baking dish and press down into an even layer. Bake in preheated oven for 15 minutes. Allow to cool before slicing into bars.
Prep Time: 10 minutes

Egg and Veggie Breakfast Sandwich:

Ingredients: 2 eggs, 2 slices whole-grain bread, 2 slices tomato, 2 slices avocado, 1/4 teaspoon sea salt, 1/4 teaspoon freshly ground black pepper

Instructions: Heat a large skillet over medium heat. Add eggs and season with salt and pepper. Cook for 3 minutes, flipping once. Place one egg on each slice of bread and top with tomato and avocado slices.

Prep Time: 5 minutes

Frittata Muffins:

Ingredients: 8 eggs, 1/4 cup diced onion, 1/4 cup diced bell pepper, 1/4 cup diced mushrooms, 1/4 cup diced ham, 1/2 teaspoon sea salt, 1/4 teaspoon freshly ground black pepper

Instructions: Preheat oven to 350°F. Grease a 12-cup muffin tin. In a large bowl, whisk together eggs, onion, bell pepper, mushrooms, ham, salt, and pepper. Pour egg mixture into muffin cups, filling each cup halfway. Bake in preheated oven for 20 minutes.

Prep Time: 10 minutes

<u>Banana Oat Muffins:</u>
Ingredients: 1 cup rolled oats, 1/4 cup almond meal, 1 teaspoon baking powder, 1 teaspoon ground cinnamon, 1/4 teaspoon sea salt, 2 ripe bananas, 1/4 cup almond butter, 1/4 cup honey
Instructions: Preheat oven to 350°F. Line a muffin tin with paper liners. In a medium bowl, combine oats, almond meal, baking powder, cinnamon, and salt. In a separate bowl, mash bananas. Add almond butter and honey and mix until combined. Add wet ingredients to dry ingredients and stir until just combined. Divide batter evenly among muffin cups and bake for 20 minutes.
Prep Time: 10 minutes

<u>Apple Cinnamon Oatmeal:</u>
Ingredients: 1 cup rolled oats, 1 cup unsweetened almond milk, 1/2 teaspoon ground cinnamon, 1/4 teaspoon sea salt, 1/4

cup chopped walnuts, 1/4 cup raisins, 1 apple, diced

Instructions: In a small saucepan, combine oats, almond milk, cinnamon, and salt. Bring to a boil, reduce heat to low, and simmer for 5 minutes. Stir in walnuts, raisins, and apple and cook for 2 minutes.

Prep Time: 10 minutes

<u>Egg and Avocado Toast:</u>

Ingredients: 2 slices whole-grain bread, 2 eggs, 1/2 avocado, sliced, 1/4 teaspoon sea salt, 1/4 teaspoon freshly ground black pepper

Instructions: Toast bread in a toaster. In a medium skillet, cook eggs for 4 minutes, flipping once. Place eggs on top of toast and top with avocado slices. Sprinkle with salt and pepper.

Prep Time: 5 minutes

<u>Coconut Chia Pudding:</u>

Ingredients: 1/2 cup chia seeds, 2 cups unsweetened coconut milk, 2 tablespoons honey, 1 teaspoon vanilla extract, 1/4 teaspoon ground cinnamon

Instructions: In a medium bowl, combine chia seeds, coconut milk, honey, vanilla extract, and cinnamon. Mix until combined. Cover and refrigerate for at least 1 hour or overnight.

Prep Time: 5 minutes

<u>Sweet Potato Toast:</u>

Ingredients: 2 sweet potatoes, 1 tablespoon olive oil, 1/2 teaspoon sea salt, 1/4 teaspoon freshly ground black pepper

Instructions: Preheat oven to 400°F. Cut sweet potatoes into 1/4-inch thick slices. Place on a baking sheet and brush with olive oil. Sprinkle with salt and pepper. Bake for 20 minutes, flipping once.

Prep Time: 10 minutes

<u>Bacon and Kale Egg Cups:</u>

Ingredients: 4 slices bacon, 4 eggs, 1/2 cup kale, chopped, 1/2 teaspoon sea salt, 1/4 teaspoon freshly ground black pepper

Instructions: Preheat oven to 350°F. Grease a 12-cup muffin tin. Cut bacon slices in half and place one half in each muffin cup. Crack one egg into each muffin cup, on top of the bacon. Top with kale and sprinkle with salt and pepper. Bake in preheated oven for 20 minutes.
Prep Time: 10 minutes

Egg and Broccoli Breakfast Bowl:
Ingredients: 2 eggs, 1 cup broccoli florets, 1 tablespoon olive oil, 1/2 teaspoon sea salt, 1/4 teaspoon freshly ground black pepper, 1/4 cup unsweetened almond milk, 1/4 cup walnuts, chopped
Instructions: Heat a large skillet over medium heat. Add olive oil, broccoli, salt, and pepper and cook for 5 minutes, stirring occasionally. Crack two eggs into the skillet and cook for 5 minutes, stirring occasionally. Place cooked broccoli and eggs in a bowl and pour almond milk over top. Top with walnuts.
Prep Time: 10 minutes

Smoked Salmon and Avocado Toast:
Ingredients: 2 slices whole-grain bread, 2 slices smoked salmon, 1/2 avocado, sliced, 1/4 teaspoon sea salt, 1/4 teaspoon freshly ground black pepper
Instructions: Toast bread in a toaster. Place smoked salmon on top of toast and top with avocado slices. Sprinkle with salt and pepper.
Prep Time: 5 minutes

Zucchini Pancakes:
Ingredients: 2 zucchini, grated, 2 eggs, 2 tablespoons almond flour, 1/2 teaspoon sea salt, 1/4 teaspoon freshly ground black pepper
Instructions: Place grated zucchini in a colander and allow to sit for 10 minutes to drain off excess water. In a medium bowl, whisk together eggs, almond flour, salt, and pepper. Add grated zucchini and mix until combined. Heat a large skillet over medium heat. Grease skillet with olive oil and drop

batter into skillet, forming pancakes. Cook for 3 minutes, flipping once.
Prep Time: 10 minutes

<u>Egg and Mushroom Breakfast Bowl:</u>
Ingredients: 2 eggs, 1/2 cup chopped mushrooms, 1 tablespoon olive oil, 1/2 teaspoon sea salt, 1/4 teaspoon freshly ground black pepper, 1/4 cup unsweetened almond milk, 1/4 cup chopped fresh parsley
Instructions: Heat a large skillet over medium heat. Add olive oil, mushrooms, salt, and pepper and cook for 5 minutes, stirring occasionally. Crack two eggs into the skillet and cook for 5 minutes, stirring occasionally. Place cooked mushrooms and eggs in a bowl and pour almond milk over top. Top with parsley.
Prep Time: 10 minutes

<u>Apple and Almond Butter Toast:</u>
Ingredients: 2 slices whole-grain bread, 1/4 cup almond butter, 1 apple, sliced

Instructions: Toast bread in a toaster. Spread almond butter on toast and top with apple slices.
Prep Time: 5 minutes

<u>Egg and Tomato Breakfast Sandwich:</u>
Ingredients: 2 eggs, 2 slices whole-grain bread, 2 slices tomato, 1/4 teaspoon sea salt, 1/4 teaspoon freshly ground black pepper
Instructions: Heat a large skillet over medium heat. Add eggs and season with salt and pepper. Cook for 3 minutes, flipping once. Place one egg on each slice of bread and top with tomato slices.
Prep Time: 5 minutes

<u>Banana Walnut Pancakes:</u>
Ingredients: 1 banana, mashed, 2 eggs, 2 tablespoons almond flour, 1/2 teaspoon baking powder, 1/2 teaspoon ground cinnamon, 1/4 teaspoon sea salt, 1/4 cup chopped walnuts
Instructions: In a medium bowl, whisk together eggs, almond flour, baking powder,

cinnamon, and salt. Add mashed banana and mix until combined. Stir in walnuts. Heat a large skillet over medium heat. Grease skillet with olive oil and drop batter into skillet, forming pancakes. Cook for 3 minutes, flipping once.
Prep Time: 10 minutes

<u>Veggie Egg Breakfast Bowl:</u>
Ingredients: 2 eggs, 1/2 cup chopped onion, 1/2 cup chopped bell pepper, 1/2 cup chopped mushrooms, 1 tablespoon olive oil, 1/2 teaspoon sea salt, 1/4 teaspoon freshly ground black pepper
Instructions: Heat a large skillet over medium heat. Add olive oil, onion, bell pepper, mushrooms, salt, and pepper and cook for 5 minutes, stirring occasionally. Crack two eggs into the skillet and cook for 5 minutes, stirring occasionally.
Prep Time: 10 minutes

<u>Blueberry Chia Pudding:</u>

Ingredients: 1/2 cup chia seeds, 2 cups unsweetened almond milk, 2 tablespoons honey, 1 teaspoon vanilla extract, 1/4 teaspoon ground cinnamon, 1/2 cup blueberries

Instructions: In a medium bowl, combine chia seeds, almond milk, honey, vanilla extract, and cinnamon. Mix until combined. Stir in blueberries. Cover and refrigerate for at least 1 hour or overnight.

Prep Time: 5 minutes

Whole30 Breakfast Burrito Bowl:

Ingredients: 2 eggs, 1/2 cup diced onion, 1/2 cup diced bell pepper, 1/2 cup diced mushrooms, 1/2 cup diced tomatoes, 1 tablespoon olive oil, 1/2 teaspoon sea salt, 1/4 teaspoon freshly ground black pepper, 1/4 cup chopped fresh cilantro

Instructions: Heat a large skillet over medium heat. Add olive oil, onion, bell pepper, mushrooms, tomatoes, salt, and pepper and cook for 5 minutes, stirring occasionally. Crack two eggs into the skillet

and cook for 5 minutes, stirring occasionally. Place cooked vegetables and eggs in a bowl and top with cilantro.
Prep Time: 10 minutes

<u>Kale, Bacon, and Egg Breakfast Bowl:</u>
Ingredients: 4 slices bacon, 4 eggs, 1 cup kale, chopped, 1/2 teaspoon sea salt, 1/4 teaspoon freshly ground black pepper, 1/4 cup unsweetened almond milk
Instructions: Preheat a large skillet over medium heat. Add bacon slices and cook for 5 minutes, flipping once. Remove bacon and set aside. In the same skillet, add eggs, kale, salt, and pepper. Cook for 5 minutes, stirring occasionally. Place cooked bacon and egg mixture in a bowl and pour almond milk over top.
Prep Time: 10 minutes

<u>Apple Cinnamon Porridge:</u>
Ingredients: 1 cup rolled oats, 2 cups unsweetened almond milk, 1 apple, diced, 1

teaspoon ground cinnamon, 1/4 teaspoon sea salt, 2 tablespoons honey

Instructions: In a medium saucepan, combine oats, almond milk, apple, cinnamon, and salt. Bring to a boil, reduce heat to low, and simmer for 5 minutes. Stir in honey.

Prep Time: 10 minutes

<u>Zucchini Omelette:</u>

Ingredients: 2 eggs, 1/2 cup grated zucchini, 1 tablespoon olive oil, 1/2 teaspoon sea salt, 1/4 teaspoon freshly ground black pepper

Instructions: Place grated zucchini in a colander and allow to sit for 10 minutes to drain off excess water. Heat a large skillet over medium heat. Add olive oil and zucchini and cook for 2 minutes. In a bowl, whisk together eggs, salt, and pepper. Pour egg mixture into skillet and cook for 5 minutes, flipping once.

Prep Time: 10 minutes

<u>Bacon, Egg, and Avocado Sandwich:</u>

Ingredients: 4 slices bacon, 4 eggs, 2 slices whole-grain bread, 1/2 avocado, sliced, 1/4 teaspoon sea salt, 1/4 teaspoon freshly ground black pepper

Instructions: Preheat a large skillet over medium heat. Add bacon slices and cook for 5 minutes, flipping once. Remove bacon and set aside. In the same skillet, add eggs, salt, and pepper. Cook for 5 minutes, flipping once. Place two bacon slices and one egg on each slice of bread and top with avocado slices.

Prep Time: 10 minutes

Sweet Potato Hash:

Ingredients: 2 sweet potatoes, 1 tablespoon olive oil, 1/2 teaspoon sea salt, 1/4 teaspoon freshly ground black pepper

Instructions: Preheat oven to 400°F. Cut sweet potatoes into cubes and place on a baking sheet. Drizzle with olive oil, salt, and pepper. Roast for 30 minutes, stirring occasionally.

Prep Time: 10 minutes

Bacon and Egg Breakfast Salad:
Ingredients: 4 slices bacon, 4 eggs, 2 cups baby spinach, 1/4 cup sliced red onion, 1/4 cup chopped cherry tomatoes, 1/4 teaspoon sea salt, 1/4 teaspoon freshly ground black pepper
Instructions: Preheat a large skillet over medium heat. Add bacon slices and cook for 5 minutes, flipping once. Remove bacon and set aside. In the same skillet, add eggs, salt, and pepper. Cook for 5 minutes, flipping once. Place bacon, eggs, spinach, onion, and tomatoes in a bowl and toss to combine.
Prep Time: 10 minutes

Egg and Asparagus Frittata:
Ingredients: 4 eggs, 1/2 cup chopped asparagus, 1 tablespoon olive oil, 1/2 teaspoon sea salt, 1/4 teaspoon freshly ground black pepper
Instructions: Preheat oven to 350°F. Heat a large skillet over medium heat. Add olive oil, asparagus, salt, and pepper and cook for 5

minutes, stirring occasionally. In a bowl, whisk together eggs. Pour egg mixture over the vegetables and cook for 5 minutes. Place skillet in preheated oven and bake for 15 minutes.
Prep Time: 10 minutes

<u>Sweet Potato Breakfast Bowl with Almonds and Blueberries:</u>
Ingredients: 2 sweet potatoes, 1 tablespoon olive oil, 1/2 teaspoon sea salt, 1/4 teaspoon freshly ground black pepper, 1/4 cup unsweetened almond milk, 1/4 cup almonds, chopped, 1/4 cup blueberries
Instructions: Preheat oven to 400°F. Cut sweet potatoes into cubes and place on a baking sheet. Drizzle with olive oil, salt, and pepper. Roast for 30 minutes, stirring occasionally. Place cooked sweet potatoes in a bowl and pour almond milk over top. Top with almonds and blueberries.
Prep Time: 10 minutes

<u>Avocado Toast with Egg and Tomato:</u>

Ingredients: 2 slices whole-grain bread, 1/2 avocado, sliced, 2 eggs, 2 slices tomato, 1/4 teaspoon sea salt, 1/4 teaspoon freshly ground black pepper
Instructions:

<u>Whole30 Baked Eggs with Bacon and Spinach:</u>
Ingredients: 6 slices bacon, diced; 1/4 onion, diced; 2 cloves garlic, minced; 1 tb spoon paprika; 2 cups spinach; 6 large eggs; 1/4 cup full-fat coconut milk; 2 tbsp olive oil
Instructions: Preheat oven to 350°F. Heat olive oil in a large skillet over medium-high heat. Add diced bacon and cook for 5 minutes, stirring occasionally. Add onion, garlic, and paprika and cook for an additional 5 minutes, stirring occasionally. Add spinach and cook for an additional 2 minutes. Divide the mixture evenly among 6 small ramekins. Crack 1 egg into each ramekin and pour 1 tablespoon of coconut

milk over the top of each. Bake for 15 minutes, until eggs are cooked through.
Prep Time: 15 minutes

<u>Whole30 Breakfast Skillet:</u>
Ingredients: 1 lb ground turkey; 1/2 onion, diced; 1 red pepper, diced; 2 cloves garlic, minced; 1 tsp chili powder; 1/2 tsp cumin; 1/4 cup full-fat coconut milk; 2 tbsp olive oil; 1/4 cup cilantro, chopped; 1 avocado, diced
Instructions: Heat olive oil in a large skillet over medium-high heat. Add ground turkey, onion, red pepper, garlic, chili powder, and cumin. Cook for 10 minutes, stirring occasionally until the turkey is cooked through. Reduce heat to low and stir in coconut milk. Serve in bowls topped with diced avocado and cilantro.
Prep Time: 15 minutes

<u>Whole30 Egg Muffins:</u>

Ingredients: 6 large eggs; 1/2 onion, diced; 1 red pepper, diced; 2 cloves garlic, minced; 1/2 tsp paprika; 1/2 tsp cumin; 2 cups spinach; 2 tbsp olive oil

Instructions: Preheat oven to 350°F. Heat olive oil in a large skillet over medium-high heat. Add onion, red pepper, garlic, paprika, and cumin. Cook for 5 minutes, stirring occasionally. Add spinach and cook for an additional 2 minutes. Divide mixture evenly among 6 greased muffin tins. Crack 1 egg into each tin. Bake for 15 minutes, until eggs are cooked through.

Prep Time: 15 minutes

<u>Whole30 Breakfast Tacos:</u>

Ingredients: 1 lb ground turkey; 1/2 onion, diced; 1 red pepper, diced; 2 cloves garlic, minced; 1 tsp chili powder; 1/2 tsp cumin; 6 small corn tortillas; 2 cups spinach; 2 tbsp olive oil; 1/4 cup cilantro, chopped

Instructions: Heat olive oil in a large skillet over medium-high heat. Add ground turkey, onion, red pepper, garlic, chili powder, and cumin. Cook for 10 minutes, stirring occasionally until the turkey is cooked through. Add spinach and cook for an additional 2 minutes. Serve in small corn tortillas topped with cilantro.

Prep Time: 15 minutes

Whole30 Breakfast Bowl with Avocado and Tomatoes:

Ingredients: 2 avocados, diced; 1/2 pint cherry tomatoes, halved; 2 cloves garlic, minced; 1/2 tsp paprika; 2 cups spinach; 2 tbsp olive oil

Instructions: Heat olive oil in a large skillet over medium-high heat. Add garlic and paprika and cook for 1 minute, stirring occasionally. Add spinach and cook for an additional 2 minutes. Serve in bowls topped with diced avocado and halved cherry tomatoes.

Prep Time: 5 minutes

Whole30 Chorizo and Egg Breakfast Casserole:

Ingredients: 1 lb chorizo sausage, cooked and crumbled; 6 large eggs; 1/2 onion, diced; 1 red pepper, diced; 2 cloves garlic, minced; 1/2 tsp paprika; 2 cups spinach; 2 tbsp olive oil

Instructions: Preheat oven to 350°F. Heat olive oil in a large skillet over medium-high heat. Add onion, red pepper, garlic, paprika, and chorizo. Cook for 5 minutes, stirring occasionally. Add spinach and cook for an additional 2 minutes. Transfer the mixture to a greased baking dish. Crack eggs over the top and bake for 20 minutes, until eggs are cooked through.

Prep Time: 10 minutes

Whole30 Breakfast Bowl with Bacon and Mushrooms:

Ingredients: 6 slices bacon, diced; 1/2 onion, diced; 1/2 lb mushrooms, sliced; 2 cloves garlic, minced; 1/2 tsp paprika; 2 cups spinach; 2 tbsp olive oil

Instructions: Heat olive oil in a large skillet over medium-high heat. Add bacon and cook for 5 minutes, stirring occasionally. Add onion, mushrooms, garlic, and paprika and cook for an additional 5 minutes, stirring occasionally. Add spinach and cook for an additional 2 minutes. Serve in bowls.
Prep Time: 10 minutes

Whole30 Breakfast Sausage:
Ingredients: 1 lb ground turkey; 1/2 onion, diced; 1 red pepper, diced; 2 cloves garlic, minced; 1 tsp chili powder; 1/2 tsp cumin; 1/4 cup full-fat coconut milk; 2 tbsp olive oil
Instructions: Heat olive oil in a large skillet over medium-high heat. Add ground turkey, onion, red pepper, garlic, chili powder, and cumin. Cook for 10 minutes, stirring occasionally until turkey is cooked through. Reduce heat to low and stir in coconut milk. Serve as is or in sandwiches or wraps.
Prep Time: 15 minutes

<u>Whole30 Breakfast Sweet Potato Skillet:</u>
Ingredients: 2 sweet potatoes, diced; 1/2 onion, diced; 2 cloves garlic, minced; 1/2 tsp paprika; 1/2 tsp cumin; 2 cups spinach; 2 tbsp olive oil
Instructions: Heat olive oil in a large skillet over medium-high heat. Add diced sweet potato and cook for 5 minutes, stirring occasionally. Add onion, garlic, paprika, and cumin and cook for an additional 5 minutes, stirring occasionally. Add spinach and cook for an additional 2 minutes. Serve in bowls.
Prep Time: 10 minutes

<u>Whole30 Egg and Tomato Breakfast Skillet:</u>
Ingredients: 6 large eggs; 1/2 onion, diced; 1 red pepper, diced; 2 cloves garlic, minced; 1/2 tsp paprika; 1/2 tsp cumin; 1/2 pint cherry tomatoes, halved; 2 cups spinach; 2 tbsp olive oil
Instructions: Heat olive oil in a large skillet over medium-high heat. Add onion, red pepper, garlic, paprika, and cumin. Cook for 5 minutes, stirring occasionally. Add

spinach and tomatoes and cook for an additional 2 minutes. Crack eggs into skillet and cook for an additional 5 minutes, stirring occasionally, until eggs are cooked through. Serve in bowls.

Prep Time: 10 minutes

<u>Whole30 Breakfast Bowl with Bacon, Mushrooms, and Avocado:</u>

Ingredients: 6 slices bacon, diced; 1/2 onion, diced; 1/2 lb mushrooms, sliced; 2 cloves garlic, minced; 1/2 tsp paprika; 2 cups spinach; 2 avocados, diced; 2 tbsp olive oil

Instructions: Heat olive oil in a large skillet over medium-high heat. Add bacon and cook for about 5 minutes until crisp. Add onion and mushrooms to the skillet and cook for about 5 minutes until softened. Add garlic and paprika and cook for an additional minute. Add spinach and cook for about 2 minutes until wilted. Divide mixture into two bowls. Top each bowl with avocado and serve. Enjoy!

<u>Chicken Cobb Salad</u>
Ingredients:
2 cups cooked chicken, shredded or diced
4 cups mixed greens
1 cup cherry tomatoes, halved
1 avocado, sliced
4 slices bacon, cooked and crumbled
2 hard-boiled eggs, sliced
1/4 cup red onion, thinly sliced
Juice of 1 lemon
2 tbsp olive oil
Salt and pepper, to taste

Instructions:
In a large bowl, combine the mixed greens, cherry tomatoes, avocado, bacon, hard-boiled eggs, and red onion.
In a separate small bowl, whisk together the lemon juice, olive oil, salt, and pepper.
Drizzle the dressing over the salad and toss to combine. Serve immediately.
Prep Time: 15 minutes

<u>Grilled Chicken and Vegetable Skewers</u>
Ingredients:
1 pound boneless, skinless chicken breasts, cut into cubes
2 bell peppers, cut into chunks
2 zucchini, cut into rounds
1 red onion, cut into chunks
2 tbsp olive oil
1 tsp garlic powder
1 tsp onion powder
1 tsp dried oregano
Salt and pepper, to taste

Instructions:
Preheat a grill or grill pan to medium-high heat.
Thread the chicken and vegetables onto skewers, alternating between the chicken and vegetables.
In a small bowl, whisk together the olive oil, garlic powder, onion powder, oregano, salt, and pepper.
Brush the skewers with the olive oil mixture.

Grill the skewers for 10-12 minutes, turning occasionally, until the chicken is cooked through and the vegetables are tender.
Prep Time: 20 minutes

Tuna Salad Lettuce Wraps
Ingredients:
2 cans tuna, drained
1/2 cup mayonnaise
1 celery stalk, diced
1/4 cup red onion, diced
1 tbsp lemon juice
Salt and pepper, to taste
Butter lettuce leaves, for serving

Instructions:
In a large bowl, mix together the tuna, mayonnaise, celery, red onion, lemon juice, salt, and pepper.
Spoon the tuna salad onto the butter lettuce leaves.
Roll the leaves up around the filling to make lettuce wraps.
Prep Time: 10 minutes

<u>Baked Sweet Potato with Chicken and Avocado</u>

Ingredients: 1 large sweet potato, 1 cup shredded chicken, 1/2 avocado, 1/4 cup chopped cilantro, 1/4 cup diced red onion, 1 tbsp. olive oil

Instructions: Preheat oven to 400°F. Pierce the sweet potato with a fork several times and bake for 45-50 minutes. Once done, slice the sweet potato in half and top each half with shredded chicken, diced avocado, cilantro, and red onion. Drizzle with olive oil.

Prep time: 10 minutes, Cook time: 45-50 minutes

Italian Turkey Skillet

Ingredients: 1 lb. ground turkey, 1 zucchini, 1 yellow squash, 1/2 onion, 1 red bell pepper, 1 can of diced tomatoes, 2 tbsp. olive oil, 1 tsp. Italian seasoning, 1/2 tsp. garlic powder, salt and pepper

Instructions: Heat olive oil in a skillet over medium-high heat. Add ground turkey and cook until browned. Add diced onion, sliced zucchini, sliced yellow squash, and diced red bell pepper. Cook for 5-7 minutes or until vegetables are tender. Add can of diced tomatoes, Italian seasoning, garlic powder, salt, and pepper. Cook for an additional 2-3 minutes.

Prep time: 10 minutes, Cook time: 20 minutes

Grilled Chicken Salad

Ingredients: 2 cups mixed greens, 1 grilled chicken breast, 1/2 avocado, 1/4 cup chopped walnuts, 1/4 cup dried cranberries, 2 tbsp. olive oil, 1 tbsp. balsamic vinegar

Instructions: Grill the chicken breast until fully cooked. Slice chicken into thin strips. Assemble mixed greens in a bowl and top with sliced chicken, diced avocado, chopped walnuts, and dried cranberries. Drizzle with olive oil and balsamic vinegar.

Prep time: 10 minutes, Cook time: 15 minutes

<u>Asian Beef Lettuce Wraps</u>
Ingredients: 1 lb. ground beef, 1/4 cup diced green onion, 1/4 cup diced water chestnuts, 1 tbsp. minced garlic, 1 tbsp. minced ginger, 1 tbsp. coconut aminos, 1 tbsp. sesame oil, 1 tbsp. olive oil, 1 head of iceberg lettuce
Instructions: Heat olive oil in a skillet over medium-high heat. Add ground beef and cook until browned. Add green onion, water chestnuts, garlic, and ginger. Cook for 3-4 minutes. Add coconut aminos and sesame oil. Cook for an additional 2-3 minutes. Spoon beef mixture onto iceberg lettuce leaves and wrap.
Prep time: 10 minutes, Cook time: 15 minutes

<u>Cucumber and Avocado Soup</u>
Ingredients: 2 ripe avocados, 1 cucumber, 1/4 cup chopped fresh dill, 2 cups vegetable broth, 1/2 cup coconut milk, 1/4 cup diced

red onion, 1/4 tsp. cayenne pepper, salt and pepper

Instructions: Peel and dice the cucumber. Add the cucumber, avocados, dill, vegetable broth, coconut milk, red onion, cayenne pepper, salt, and pepper to a blender. Blend until smooth. Serve chilled.

Prep time: 10 minutes

<u>Zucchini Noodle Stir Fry with Sesame-Ginger Sauce</u>
Ingredients:
- 2 tablespoons sesame oil
- 1 red bell pepper, julienned
- 1 yellow bell pepper, julienned
- 1 cup mushrooms, sliced
- 1 bunch of scallions, diced
- 2 cloves garlic, minced
- 2 zucchinis, spiralized into noodles
- 2 tablespoons coconut aminos
- 2 tablespoons rice vinegar
- 1 teaspoon grated ginger
- 2 tablespoons sesame seeds

Instructions:
1. Heat the sesame oil in a large skillet over medium heat.
2. Add the bell peppers, mushrooms, scallions, and garlic and sauté for 5 minutes, until the vegetables are softened.

3. Add the zucchini noodles and sauté for an additional 3 minutes.
4. In a small bowl, whisk together the coconut aminos, rice vinegar, and ginger.
5. Pour the mixture over the vegetables and noodles and cook for an additional 2 minutes.
6. Sprinkle with sesame seeds and serve.

Preparation Method: Sauté
Prep Time: 10 minutes

<u>Baked Salmon with Citrus and Herbs</u>
Ingredients:
- 2 salmon fillets
- 2 tablespoons olive oil
- Juice of 1 lemon
- 1 teaspoon fresh rosemary, chopped
- 1 teaspoon fresh thyme, chopped
- 1 teaspoon fresh oregano, chopped
- 1 teaspoon garlic powder
- Salt and pepper, to taste

Instructions:

1. Preheat oven to 375°F.
2. Place the salmon fillets on a greased baking sheet.
3. In a small bowl, mix the olive oil, lemon juice, rosemary, thyme, oregano, garlic powder, salt, and pepper.
4. Brush the salmon with the mixture.
5. Bake for 15-20 minutes, or until the salmon is cooked through.

Preparation Method: Bake
Prep Time: 15-20 minutes

<u>Sautéed Pork Chops with Apples and Onions</u>
<u>Ingredients:</u>
- 2 tablespoons olive oil
- 2 pork chops
- 1 onion, sliced
- 1 apple, sliced
- 1 teaspoon garlic powder
- 1 teaspoon smoked paprika
- Salt and pepper, to taste

Instructions:

1. Heat the olive oil in a large skillet over medium heat.
2. Add the pork chops and cook for 3-4 minutes per side, until golden brown.
3. Add the onion and apple and sauté for an additional 5 minutes.
4. Sprinkle with garlic powder, smoked paprika, salt, and pepper.
5. Continue to cook for an additional 5 minutes, or until the pork chops are cooked through and the vegetables are softened.

Preparation Method: Sauté
Prep Time: 15 minutes

Cauliflower Rice Burrito Bowls
Ingredients:
- 2 tablespoons olive oil
- 1 head cauliflower, grated
- 1 tablespoon chili powder
- 1 teaspoon cumin
- 1 can black beans, drained and rinsed
- 1 cup cherry tomatoes, halved
- ½ cup cilantro, chopped

- Juice of 1 lime
- Salt and pepper, to taste

Instructions:
1. Heat the olive oil in a large skillet over medium heat.
2. Add the grated cauliflower and sauté for 5 minutes, until softened.
3. Add the chili powder and cumin and cook for an additional 1 minute.
4. Add the black beans, cherry tomatoes, cilantro, lime juice, salt, and pepper and cook for an additional 3 minutes.
5. Serve in bowls and enjoy.

Preparation Method: Sauté
Prep Time: 10 minutes

Roasted Sweet Potato and Kale Salad
Ingredients:
- 2 sweet potatoes, cubed
- 2 tablespoons olive oil
- 1 teaspoon garlic powdcr
- 1 teaspoon dried oregano

- Salt and pepper, to taste
- 4 cups kale, chopped
- ½ cup dried cranberries
- ¼ cup walnuts, chopped
- 2 tablespoons balsamic vinegar

Instructions:
1. Preheat oven to 375°F.
2. Place the cubed sweet potatoes on a greased baking sheet and toss with the olive oil, garlic powder, oregano, salt, and pepper.
3. Roast for 20 minutes, or until the potatoes are tender.
4. In a large bowl, combine the roasted sweet potatoes, kale, cranberries, walnuts, and balsamic vinegar.
5. Toss to combine and serve.

Preparation Method: Roast
Prep Time: 25 minutes

<u>Coconut-Lime Chicken</u>
Ingredients:
- 2 tablespoons coconut oil

- 2 boneless, skinless chicken breasts
- Juice of 1 lime
- 2 tablespoons coconut milk
- 2 cloves garlic, minced
- 1 teaspoon grated ginger
- 2 tablespoons chopped cilantro
- Salt and pepper, to taste

Instructions:
1. Heat the coconut oil in a large skillet over medium heat.
2. Add the chicken and cook for 3-4 minutes per side, until cooked through.
3. In a small bowl, whisk together the lime juice, coconut milk, garlic, ginger, cilantro, salt, and pepper.
4. Pour the mixture over the chicken and cook for an additional 2 minutes.
5. Serve and enjoy.

Preparation Method: Sauté
Prep Time: 10 minutes

Eggplant and Bell Pepper Ratatouille

Ingredients:
- 2 tablespoons olive oil
- 1 eggplant, cubed
- 1 red bell pepper, cubed
- 1 yellow bell pepper, cubed
- 1 onion, diced
- 2 cloves garlic, minced
- 2 tablespoons tomato paste
- 1 can diced tomatoes
- Salt and pepper, to taste

Instructions:
1. Heat the olive oil in a large skillet over medium heat.
2. Add the eggplant, bell peppers, onion, and garlic and sauté for 5 minutes, until the vegetables are softened.
3. Add the tomato paste and diced tomatoes and cook for an additional 5 minutes.
4. Season with salt and pepper.
5. Serve and enjoy.

Preparation Method: Sauté
Prep Time: 10 minutes

Grilled Chicken Skewers with Pineapple

Ingredients:

- 2 boneless, skinless chicken breasts, cut into cubes
- 2 tablespoons olive oil
- Juice of 1 lime
- 1 teaspoon garlic powder
- ½ teaspoon chili powder
- ½ teaspoon smoked paprika
- 1 teaspoon honey
- ½ pineapple, cut into cubes

Instructions:

1. Preheat the grill to medium-high heat.
2. Thread the chicken and pineapple onto skewers.
3. In a small bowl, mix the olive oil, lime juice, garlic powder, chili powder, smoked paprika, and honey.
4. Brush the marinade over the chicken and pineapple skewers.
5. Grill for 5-7 minutes per side, or until the chicken is cooked through.

Preparation Method: Grill
Prep Time: 10 minutes

<u>Baked Cod with Tomatoes and Olives</u>
Ingredients:
- 2 cod fillets
- 2 tablespoons olive oil
- 2 cloves garlic, minced
- 2 cups cherry tomatoes, halved
- ½ cup kalamata olives, halved
- Juice of 1 lemon
- 2 tablespoons fresh parsley, chopped
- Salt and pepper, to taste

Instructions:
1. Preheat oven to 375°F.
2. Place the cod fillets in a greased baking dish.
3. In a small bowl, mix the olive oil, garlic, cherry tomatoes, olives, lemon juice, parsley, salt, and pepper.
4. Pour the mixture over the cod fillets.

5. Bake for 15-20 minutes, or until the cod is cooked through.

Preparation Method: Bake
Prep Time: 15-20 minutes

<u>Sautéed Brussels Sprouts with Bacon</u>
Ingredients:
- 2 tablespoons olive oil
- 2 cups Brussels sprouts, halved
- 4 slices bacon, cooked and chopped
- 1 shallot, minced
- 1 teaspoon garlic powder
- 2 tablespoons balsamic vinegar
- Salt and pepper, to taste

Instructions:
1. Heat the olive oil in a large skillet over medium heat.
2. Add the Brussels sprouts and sauté for 5 minutes, until softened.
3. Add the bacon, shallot, garlic powder, and balsamic vinegar and cook for an additional 3 minutes.

4. Season with salt and pepper.
5. Serve and enjoy.

Preparation Method: Sauté
Prep Time: 10 minutes

<u>Steak Fajitas</u>
Ingredients:
- 2 tablespoons olive oil
- 2 steak fillets
- 1 red bell pepper, julienned
- 1 yellow bell pepper, julienned
- 1 onion, sliced
- 1 teaspoon chili powder
- 1 teaspoon garlic powder
- Juice of 1 lime
- Salt and pepper, to taste

Instructions:
1. Heat the olive oil in a large skillet over medium heat.
2. Add the steak and cook for 3-4 minutes per side, until cooked through.

3. Remove the steak from the skillet and set aside.

4. Add the bell peppers and onion and sauté for 5 minutes, until softened.

5. Add the chili powder, garlic powder, lime juice, salt, and pepper and cook for an additional 3 minutes.

6. Slice the steak and add it back to the skillet.

7. Serve with your favorite toppings and enjoy.

Preparation Method: Sauté
Prep Time: 15 minutes

Baked Sweet Potato Hash
Ingredients:
- 2 tablespoons olive oil
- 1 onion, diced
- 2 sweet potatoes, cubed
- 1 teaspoon garlic powder
- 1 teaspoon smoked paprika
- 2 tablespoons chopped fresh rosemary
- Salt and pepper, to taste

Instructions:
1. Preheat oven to 375°F.
2. Heat the olive oil in a large skillet over medium heat.
3. Add the onion and sweet potatoes and sauté for 5 minutes, until the vegetables are softened.
4. Add the garlic powder, smoked paprika, rosemary, salt, and pepper and cook for an additional 3 minutes.
5. Transfer the mixture to a greased baking dish and bake for 20 minutes, or until the sweet potatoes are tender.

Preparation Method: Bake
Prep Time: 25 minutes

Roasted Broccoli and Carrots
Ingredients:
- 2 tablespoons olive oil
- 2 cups broccoli florets
- 2 carrots, sliced
- 1 teaspoon garlic powder

- 1 teaspoon dried oregano
- Salt and pepper, to taste

Instructions:
1. Preheat oven to 375°F.
2. Place the broccoli and carrots on a greased baking sheet and toss with the olive oil, garlic powder, oregano, salt, and pepper.
3. Roast for 20 minutes, or until the vegetables are tender.
4. Serve and enjoy.

Preparation Method: Roast
Prep Time: 20 minutes

<u>Spicy Sausage and Shrimp Skillet</u>
Ingredients:
- 2 tablespoons olive oil
- 8 ounces spicy sausage, sliced
- 1 onion, diced
- 1 bell pepper, diced
- 2 cloves garlic, minced
- 8 ounces shrimp, peeled and deveined
- 2 tablespoons tomato paste

- ½ teaspoon red pepper flakes
- Salt and pepper, to taste

Instructions:
1. Heat the olive oil in a large skillet over medium heat.
2. Add the sausage and cook for 3-4 minutes, until browned.
3. Add the onion, bell pepper, and garlic and sauté for an additional 5 minutes.
4. Add the shrimp and cook for 2 minutes, until just cooked through.
5. Stir in the tomato paste and season with red pepper flakes, salt, and pepper.
6. Serve and enjoy.

Preparation Method: Sauté
Prep Time: 15 minutes

<u>Roasted Cauliflower and Chickpea Tacos</u>
Ingredients:
- 2 tablespoons olive oil
- 1 head cauliflower, cut into florets
- 1 teaspoon garlic powder

- 1 teaspoon chili powder
- 1 teaspoon smoked paprika
- 1 can chickpeas, drained and rinsed
- Salt and pepper, to taste
- 8 taco shells
- Toppings of your choice

Instructions:
1. Preheat oven to 375°F.
2. Place the cauliflower florets on a greased baking sheet and toss them with olive oil, garlic powder, chili powder, smoked paprika, salt, and pepper.
3. Roast for 20 minutes, or until the cauliflower is tender.
4. Add the chickpeas and continue to roast for an additional 5 minutes.
5. Serve the roasted cauliflower and chickpeas in taco shells with your favorite toppings.

Preparation Method: Roast
Prep Time: 25 minutes

<u>Thai Chicken Curry</u>

Ingredients:
- 2 tablespoons coconut oil
- 2 boneless, skinless chicken breasts, cubed
- 1 onion, diced
- 1 red bell pepper, diced
- 1 can of coconut milk
- 2 tablespoons red curry paste
- 2 tablespoons fish sauce
- 2 tablespoons lime juice
- 2 tablespoons chopped fresh cilantro
- Salt and pepper, to taste

Instructions:
1. Heat the coconut oil in a large skillet over medium heat.
2. Add the chicken and cook for 3-4 minutes, until cooked through.
3. Add the onion and bell pepper and sauté for an additional 5 minutes.
4. Add the coconut milk, red curry paste, fish sauce, lime juice, cilantro, salt, and pepper.

5. Simmer for 10 minutes, or until the sauce has thickened.
6. Serve and enjoy.

Preparation Method: Sauté
Prep Time: 15 minutes

<u>Baked Chicken Thighs with Rosemary and Garlic</u>
Ingredients:
- 2 tablespoons olive oil
- 4 bone-in chicken thighs
- 2 cloves garlic, minced
- 2 tablespoons fresh rosemary, chopped
- Juice of 1 lemon
- Salt and pepper, to taste

Instructions:
1. Preheat oven to 375°F.
2. Place the chicken thighs on a greased baking sheet and brush them with the olive oil.
3. Sprinkle with the garlic, rosemary, lemon juice, salt, and pepper.

4. Bake for 25-30 minutes, or until the chicken is cooked through.

Preparation Method: Bake
Prep Time: 25-30 minutes

Zucchini Noodle Pad Thai
Ingredients:
- 2 tablespoons sesame oil
- 2 zucchinis, spiralized into noodles
- 2 cloves garlic, minced
- 1 tablespoon grated ginger
- 1 red bell pepper, julienned
- ½ cup carrots, julienned
- 2 tablespoons coconut aminos
- 2 tablespoons rice vinegar
- 1 tablespoon honey
- 2 tablespoons chopped peanuts
- 2 tablespoons chopped cilantro

Instructions:
1. Heat the sesame oil in a large skillet over medium heat.

2. Add the zucchini noodles, garlic, ginger, bell pepper, and carrots and sauté for 5 minutes, until the vegetables are softened.
3. In a small bowl, whisk together the coconut aminos, rice vinegar, and honey.
4. Pour the mixture over the vegetables and noodles and cook for an additional 2 minutes.
5. Sprinkle with peanuts and cilantro and serve.

Preparation Method: Sauté
Prep Time: 10 minutes

Slow Cooker Beef Stew
Ingredients:
2 lbs beef stew meat, cut into bite-size pieces
3 carrots, chopped
3 stalks celery, chopped
1 onion, chopped
3 cloves garlic, minced
2 cups beef broth
1 tsp dried thyme
Salt and pepper to taste

Instructions:

Add beef, carrots, celery, onion, garlic, beef broth, thyme, salt, and pepper to a slow cooker.
Cover and cook on low for 6-8 hours or until beef is tender.
Prep Time: 15 minutes | Cook Time: 6-8 hours | Total Time: 6 hours 15 minutes to 8 hours 15 minutes

Grilled Lemon and Herb Chicken
Ingredients:
4 boneless, skinless chicken breasts
2 tbsp olive oil
2 tbsp fresh lemon juice
1 tbsp fresh chopped herbs (such as thyme, rosemary, and oregano)
Salt and pepper to taste
Instructions:

In a small bowl, whisk together olive oil, lemon juice, and herbs.

Season chicken with salt and pepper, then brush with the lemon herb mixture.
Grill chicken over medium-high heat for 6-7 minutes per side or until cooked through.
Serve with your favorite roasted vegetables.
Prep time: 10 minutes
Cook time: 15 minutes

<u>Spicy Shrimp Stir Fry</u>
Ingredients:
1 lb raw shrimp, peeled and deveined
1 red bell pepper, sliced
1 yellow onion, sliced
2 garlic cloves, minced
1 tbsp grated ginger
2 tbsp coconut aminos
1 tbsp sriracha sauce
Salt and pepper to taste
2 tbsp avocado oil
Instructions:

In a large skillet or wok, heat avocado oil over high heat.

Add shrimp, bell pepper, onion, garlic, and ginger to the skillet.
Cook until shrimp is pink and vegetables are tender, stirring frequently.
In a small bowl, whisk together coconut aminos and sriracha sauce. Pour over the stir fry and toss to coat.
Season with salt and pepper to taste.
Serve hot over cauliflower rice.
Prep time: 15 minutes
Cook time: 10 minutes

<u>One-Pan Chicken and Roasted Vegetables</u>
Ingredients:
4 boneless, skinless chicken breasts
1 lb Brussels sprouts, trimmed and halved
2 cups baby carrots
2 tbsp olive oil
1 tbsp dried oregano
Salt and pepper to taste
Instructions:

Preheat oven to 400°F.

In a large bowl, toss together chicken, Brussels sprouts, carrots, olive oil, oregano, salt, and pepper.
Arrange chicken and vegetables on a large baking sheet.
Bake for 25-30 minutes or until chicken is cooked through and vegetables are tender.
Serve hot.
Prep time: 15 minutes
Cook time: 30 minutes

Baked Sweet Potato Fries – Ingredients: 2 large sweet potatoes, peeled and cut into fries, 2 tablespoons olive oil, 1 teaspoon garlic powder, 1 teaspoon smoked paprika, ½ teaspoon sea salt, ½ teaspoon black pepper. Instructions: Preheat oven to 400 degrees F. In a large bowl, toss together sweet potatoes, olive oil, garlic powder, smoked paprika, sea salt, and black pepper. Spread sweet potatoes out on a baking sheet and bake for 25-30 minutes, flipping halfway through. Prep Time: 10 minutes

Cauliflower Rice – Ingredients: 1 head of cauliflower, 2 tablespoons olive oil, 1 teaspoon garlic powder, 1 teaspoon smoked paprika, ½ teaspoon sea salt, ½ teaspoon black pepper. Instructions: Cut the cauliflower into florets and place in a food processor and pulse until it is in small rice-like pieces. Heat olive oil in a large skillet over medium-high heat and add the cauliflower rice. Add the garlic powder, smoked paprika, sea salt, and black pepper and stir to combine. Cook for 5-7 minutes, stirring occasionally until the cauliflower is cooked through. Prep Time: 10 minutes

<u>Baked Apple Chips</u> – Ingredients: 2 apples, peeled and thinly sliced, 2 tablespoons coconut oil, 1 teaspoon cinnamon, 1 teaspoon nutmeg, ½ teaspoon sea salt. Instructions: Preheat oven to 250 degrees F. Line a baking sheet with parchment paper. In a large bowl, combine apples, coconut oil, cinnamon, nutmeg, and sea salt. Toss to combine. Place apple slices on the prepared baking sheet in a single layer. Bake for 1 hour, flipping the chips halfway through. Allow chips to cool before serving. Prep Time: 10 minutes

Almond Butter Fudge – Ingredients: 1 cup almond butter, ½ cup coconut oil, ¼ cup honey, 1 teaspoon vanilla extract. Instructions: Line an 8x8-inch pan with parchment paper. In a small saucepan over low heat, melt together almond butter and coconut oil until smooth. Remove from heat and stir in honey and vanilla extract. Pour mixture into prepared pan and spread evenly. Place in the refrigerator for 1-2 hours, until firm. Cut into squares and enjoy. Prep Time: 10 minutes

Roasted Nuts – Ingredients: 2 cups of raw nuts (almonds, walnuts, pecans, etc.), 2 tablespoons melted coconut oil, 1 teaspoon sea salt, ½ teaspoon garlic powder. Instructions: Preheat oven to 350 degrees F. Spread nuts out on a baking sheet. Drizzle coconut oil over nuts and sprinkle with sea salt and garlic powder. Mix everything to evenly coat the nuts. Bake for 8-10 minutes, stirring once halfway through. Allow cooling before enjoying. Prep Time: 10 minutes

<u>Coconut Date Balls</u> – Ingredients: 1 cup pitted dates, ½ cup shredded coconut, 2 tablespoons almond butter, 2 tablespoons chia seeds, 1 teaspoon vanilla extract. Instructions: Place dates in a food processor and pulse until it forms a paste. Add in shredded coconut, almond butter, chia seeds, and vanilla extract. Pulse again until everything is combined. Scoop out tablespoon-sized portions and roll them into a ball. Place in the refrigerator or freezer to firm up. Enjoy! Prep Time: 10 minutes

<u>Baked Asparagus</u> – Ingredients: 1 lb asparagus, 1 tablespoon olive oil, 1 teaspoon garlic powder, 1 teaspoon dried oregano, 1 teaspoon smoked paprika, ½ teaspoon sea salt, ½ teaspoon black pepper. Instructions: Preheat oven to 400 degrees F. Place asparagus on a baking sheet and drizzle with olive oil. Sprinkle with garlic powder, dried oregano, smoked paprika, sea salt, and black pepper. Toss to coat. Bake for 15-20

minutes, or until the asparagus is tender. Prep Time: 10 minutes

<u>Cucumber Tomato Salad</u> – Ingredients: 2 large cucumbers, diced, 2 ripe tomatoes, diced, 1 tablespoon olive oil, 1 teaspoon apple cider vinegar, ½ teaspoon sea salt, ½ teaspoon black pepper. Instructions: In a large bowl, combine cucumbers and tomatoes. Drizzle with olive oil and apple cider vinegar and season with sea salt and black pepper. Toss to combine. Enjoy! Prep Time: 10 minutes

<u>Roasted Garlic & Herb Sweet Potatoes</u> – Ingredients: 2 large sweet potatoes, peeled and cubed, 2 tablespoons olive oil, 1 teaspoon garlic powder, 1 teaspoon dried oregano, ½ teaspoon sea salt, ½ teaspoon black pepper. Instructions: Preheat oven to 400 degrees F. Place sweet potatoes on a baking sheet and drizzle with olive oil. Sprinkle with garlic powder, dried oregano, sea salt, and black pepper. Toss to coat.

Bake for 25-30 minutes, or until sweet potatoes are tender. Enjoy! Prep Time: 10 minutes

Avocado Toast – Ingredients: 2 slices of sprouted whole grain bread, 1 ripe avocado, ½ teaspoon sea salt, ½ teaspoon black pepper. Instructions: Toast bread to the desired doneness. In a small bowl, mash avocado until smooth. Spread mashed avocado on toast and season with sea salt and black pepper. Enjoy! Prep Time: 5 minutes

Zucchini Fritters – Ingredients: 2 zucchinis, grated, 2 tablespoons almond meal, 2 tablespoons coconut flour, 1 teaspoon garlic powder, 1 teaspoon dried oregano, 1 teaspoon smoked paprika, ½ teaspoon sea salt, ½ teaspoon black pepper. Instructions: In a medium bowl, combine grated zucchini, almond meal, coconut flour, garlic powder, dried oregano, smoked paprika, sea salt, and black pepper. Mix until combined. Heat a large skillet over medium-high heat and add a few tablespoons of olive oil. Scoop out 2-3 tablespoon-sized portions of the mixture and flatten into patties. Cook for 2-3 minutes on each side, or until golden brown. Enjoy! Prep Time: 10 minutes

<u>Baked Beet Chips</u> – Ingredients: 2 large beets, peeled and sliced into thin rounds, 2 tablespoons olive oil, 1 teaspoon garlic powder, 1 teaspoon smoked paprika, ½ teaspoon sea salt, ½ teaspoon black pepper. Instructions: Preheat oven to 400 degrees F. Line a baking sheet with parchment paper. Place beet slices on the prepared baking sheet and drizzle with olive oil. Sprinkle with garlic powder, smoked paprika, sea salt, and black pepper. Toss to coat. Bake for 15-20 minutes, flipping the chips halfway through. Allow cooling before serving. Prep Time: 10 minutes

<u>Egg Muffins</u> – Ingredients: 6 large eggs, ½ cup diced bell peppers, ½ cup diced onions,

½ cup diced mushrooms, ½ cup diced spinach, 2 tablespoons olive oil, 1 teaspoon garlic powder, 1 teaspoon dried oregano, 1 teaspoon smoked paprika, ½ teaspoon sea salt, ½ teaspoon black pepper. Instructions: Preheat oven to 375 degrees F. Grease a 12-cup muffin tin with olive oil. In a large bowl, whisk together eggs. Add bell peppers, onions, mushrooms, and spinach and mix to combine. Divide the mixture evenly among the muffin cups. Top with olive oil, garlic powder, dried oregano, smoked paprika, sea salt, and black pepper. Bake for 20-25 minutes, or until muffins are cooked through. Enjoy! Prep Time: 10 minutes

Celery and Hummus – Ingredients: 2 celery stalks, 1/4 cup hummus, 1 teaspoon sesame seeds, 1 teaspoon ground cumin. Instructions: Cut celery stalks into 3-4 inch pieces. Spread hummus onto the celery and sprinkle with sesame seeds and ground cumin. Enjoy! Prep Time: 5 minutes

Coconut Yogurt – Ingredients: 1 13.5-ounce can full-fat coconut milk, 2 tablespoons maple syrup, 2 tablespoons probiotic powder. Instructions: In a medium bowl, whisk together coconut milk, maple syrup, and probiotic powder until combined. Pour the mixture into a glass jar and cover it with a lid. Place jar in a warm spot and allow to sit for 12-24 hours. Refrigerate for at least 4 hours before serving. Enjoy! Prep Time: 10 minutes

Baked Plantains – Ingredients: 2 large plantains, 1 tablespoon olive oil, 1 teaspoon garlic powder, 1 teaspoon smoked paprika, ½ teaspoon sea salt, ½ teaspoon black pepper. Instructions: Preheat oven to 400 degrees F. Peel plantains and cut them into 1-inch slices. Place plantains on a baking sheet and drizzle with olive oil. Sprinkle with garlic powder, smoked paprika, sea salt, and black pepper. Toss to coat. Bake for 15-20 minutes, flipping the slices halfway through. Enjoy! Prep Time: 10 minutes

Chia Pudding – Ingredients: 1 cup almond milk, 2 tablespoons chia seeds, 1 teaspoon vanilla extract, 1 teaspoon maple syrup. Instructions: In a medium bowl, combine almond milk, chia seeds, vanilla extract, and maple syrup. Whisk until combined. Cover and refrigerate for at least 4 hours. Enjoy! Prep Time: 5 minutes

Roasted Brussels Sprouts – Ingredients: 2 cups Brussels sprouts, halved, 2 tablespoons olive oil, 1 teaspoon garlic powder, 1 teaspoon smoked paprika, ½ teaspoon sea salt, ½ teaspoon black pepper. Instructions: Preheat oven to 400 degrees F. Place Brussels sprouts on a baking sheet and drizzles with olive oil. Sprinkle with garlic powder, smoked paprika, sea salt, and black pepper. Toss to coat. Bake for 25-30 minutes, or until Brussels sprouts are tender. Enjoy! Prep Time: 10 minutes

<u>Tuna Salad</u> – Ingredients: 1 can of tuna, drained and flaked, 2 tablespoons diced celery, 2 tablespoons diced onion, 2 tablespoons diced bell pepper, 2 tablespoons diced cucumber, 2 tablespoons olive oil, 1 teaspoon apple cider vinegar, 1 teaspoon Dijon mustard, ½ teaspoon sea salt, ½ teaspoon black pepper. Instructions: In a medium bowl, combine tuna, celery, onion, bell pepper, and cucumber. Drizzle with olive oil, apple cider vinegar, and Dijon mustard. Season with sea salt and black pepper. Toss to combine. Enjoy! Prep Time: 10 minutes

<u>Almond Butter Banana Toast</u> – Ingredients: 2 slices of sprouted whole grain bread, 2 tablespoons almond butter, 1 ripe banana, sliced, 1 teaspoon cinnamon. Instructions: Toast bread to the desired doneness. Spread almond butter onto toast and top with banana slices. Sprinkle with cinnamon. Enjoy! Prep Time: 5 minutes

<u>Spicy Roasted Chickpeas</u> – Ingredients: 2 cans of chickpeas, drained and rinsed, 2 tablespoons olive oil, 1 teaspoon garlic powder, 1 teaspoon smoked paprika, 1 teaspoon chili powder, ½ teaspoon sea salt, ½ teaspoon black pepper. Instructions: Preheat oven to 400 degrees F. Place chickpeas on a baking sheet and drizzle with olive oil. Sprinkle with garlic powder, smoked paprika, chili powder, sea salt, and black pepper. Toss to coat. Bake for 25-30 minutes, or until chickpeas are crispy. Enjoy! Prep Time: 10 minutes

<u>Cucumber-Avocado Salad</u> – Ingredients: 2 large cucumbers, diced, 1 ripe avocado, diced, 2 tablespoons olive oil, 1 teaspoon lime juice, ½ teaspoon sea salt, ½ teaspoon black pepper. Instructions: In a large bowl, combine cucumbers and avocado. Drizzle with olive oil and lime juice and season with sea salt and black pepper. Toss to combine. Enjoy! Prep Time: 10 minutes

Baked Sweet Potato Chips – Ingredients: 2 large sweet potatoes, peeled and sliced into thin rounds, 2 tablespoons olive oil, 1 teaspoon garlic powder, 1 teaspoon smoked paprika, ½ teaspoon sea salt, ½ teaspoon black pepper. Instructions: Preheat oven to 400 degrees F. Line a baking sheet with parchment paper. Place sweet potato slices on the prepared baking sheet and drizzle with olive oil. Sprinkle with garlic powder, smoked paprika, sea salt, and black pepper. Toss to coat. Bake for 15-20 minutes, flipping the chips halfway through. Allow cooling before serving. Prep Time: 10 minutes

Carrot Celery Sticks – Ingredients: 2 large carrots, peeled and cut into sticks, 2 celery stalks, cut into sticks, 2 tablespoons olive oil, 1 teaspoon garlic powder, ½ teaspoon sea salt, ½ teaspoon black pepper. Instructions: Preheat oven to 400 degrees F. Place carrots and celery on a baking sheet and drizzle with olive oil. Sprinkle with garlic powder, sea salt, and black pepper. Toss to coat. Bake for 10-15 minutes, or until carrots and celery are tender. Enjoy! Prep Time: 10 minutes

<u>Kale Chips</u> – Ingredients: 2 cups of kale, 2 tablespoons olive oil, 1 teaspoon garlic powder, 1 teaspoon smoked paprika, ½ teaspoon sea salt, ½ teaspoon black pepper. Instructions: Preheat oven to 350 degrees F. Line a baking sheet with parchment paper. Place kale on the prepared baking sheet and drizzle with olive oil. Sprinkle with garlic powder, smoked paprika, sea salt, and black pepper. Toss to coat. Bake for 10-12 minutes, or until kale is crispy. Enjoy! Prep Time: 10 minutes

<u>Apple Cinnamon Chips</u>
2 large apples
1 teaspoon ground cinnamon
Preheat oven to 200°F (93°C).
Slice apples thinly and sprinkle cinnamon on top.

Place slices on a baking sheet lined with parchment paper.
Bake for 2-3 hours until crispy.
Prep time: 10 minutes.
Homemade Beef Jerky
1 lb grass-fed beef
1/4 cup coconut aminos
1/4 cup apple cider vinegar
1 tablespoon garlic powder
1 tablespoon onion powder
1/2 teaspoon smoked paprika

Instructions:
Preheat oven to 170°F (77°C).
Mix all ingredients in a bowl and let the beef marinate for at least 30 minutes.
Place beef slices on a baking sheet lined with parchment paper.
Bake for 3-4 hours until the beef is dry and chewy.
Prep time: 40 minutes.

<u>Sweet Potato Fries</u>
2 large sweet potatoes

2 tablespoons olive oil
1/2 teaspoon sea salt

Instructions:
Preheat oven to 425°F (218°C).
Cut sweet potatoes into thin fries.
Toss with olive oil and sea salt.
Place on a baking sheet lined with parchment paper.
Bake for 25-30 minutes until crispy.
Prep time: 10 minutes.

Smoked Salmon Cucumber Bites
Ingredients:
1 cucumber
4 oz smoked salmon
2 tbsp paleo mayonnaise
1 tsp dill

Instructions:
Slice the cucumber into thin rounds.
Top each cucumber slice with a small piece of smoked salmon.

In a small bowl, mix the mayonnaise and dill.
Drizzle the mayo mixture over the salmon-cucumber bites.
Prep Time: 10 minutes

<u>Deviled Eggs with Bacon</u>
Ingredients:
6 hard-boiled eggs
2 tbsp paleo mayonnaise
1 tsp dijon mustard
Salt and pepper to taste
2 slices of cooked bacon, crumbled

Instructions:
Cut the hard-boiled eggs in half and remove the yolks.
In a small bowl, mix the egg yolks, mayonnaise, dijon mustard, salt, and pepper.
Spoon the egg yolk mixture back into the egg whites.
Sprinkle crumbled bacon on top of each deviled egg.

Prep Time: 15 minutes

Grilled Pineapple Spears
Ingredients:
1 pineapple
2 tbsp coconut oil

Instructions:
Preheat a grill to medium heat.
Cut the pineapple into spears.
Brush the pineapple spears with melted coconut oil.
Grill the pineapple for 3-4 minutes on each side, until caramelized.
Prep Time: 10 minutes
Cook Time: 8-10 minutes

Antipasto Skewers
Ingredients:
12 cherry tomatoes
12 olives
12 slices of salami
12 small cubes of compliant cheese (optional)

12 small cubes of bell pepper

Instructions:
Thread a cherry tomato, olive, slice of salami, cheese (if using), and bell pepper onto each skewer.
Serve chilled.
Prep Time: 10 minutes

<u>Almond Joy Bites:</u>
Ingredients:
-1/4 cup coconut flakes
-1/4 cup slivered almonds
-2 tablespoons almond butter
-2 tablespoons honey
-1/2 teaspoon almond extract

Instructions:
1. In a medium bowl, combine coconut flakes, slivered almonds, almond butter, honey, and almond extract.
2. Mix until thoroughly combined.
3. Roll into small balls and place on a parchment-lined baking sheet.
4. Freeze for 1 hour.
Prep Time: 10 minutes

<u>Coconut Cashew Bites:</u>
Ingredients:
-1/2 cup coconut flakes

-1/2 cup raw cashews
-1/4 cup honey
-1/4 teaspoon coconut oil

Instructions:
1. In a food processor, pulse coconut flakes and cashews until they're combined.
2. Add honey and coconut oil and blend until mixed.
3. Line a baking sheet with parchment paper and scoop the mixture onto it.
4. Using your hands, shape into small bite-sized balls and place them back on the parchment paper.
5. Freeze for 1 hour.
Prep Time: 10 minutes

<u>Apple Cinnamon Bites:</u>
Ingredients:
-1 cup applesauce
-2 tablespoons maple syrup
-1 teaspoon cinnamon
-1/2 cup coconut flakes

Instructions:

1. In a medium bowl, combine applesauce, maple syrup, and cinnamon.

2. Add in the coconut flakes and mix until combined.

3. Scoop mixture onto a parchment-lined baking sheet and shape into small balls.

4. Freeze for 1 hour.

Prep Time: 10 minutes

<u>Banana Almond Bites</u>:

Ingredients:

-2 mashed bananas

-2 tablespoons almond butter

-2 tablespoons honey

-1/4 cup almond meal

Instructions:

1. In a medium bowl, combine mashed bananas, almond butter, honey, and almond meal.

2. Mix until thoroughly combined.

3. Roll into small balls and place on a parchment-lined baking sheet.

4. Freeze for 1 hour.

Prep Time: 10 minutes

<u>Chocolate Coconut Bites:</u>
Ingredients:
-1/4 cup cocoa powder
-1/4 cup coconut flakes
-1/4 cup almond butter
-2 tablespoons honey

Instructions:
1. In a medium bowl, combine cocoa powder, coconut flakes, almond butter, and honey.
2. Mix until thoroughly combined.
3. Roll into small balls and place on a parchment-lined baking sheet.
4. Freeze for 1 hour.
Prep Time: 10 minutes

<u>Date Pecan Bites:</u>
Ingredients:
-1/2 cup pitted dates
-1/4 cup pecans
-1/4 cup almond butter

-2 tablespoons honey

Instructions:
1. In a food processor, pulse dates and pecans until they're combined.
2. Add almond butter and honey and mix until combincd.
3. Line a baking sheet with parchment paper and scoop the mixture onto it.
4. Using your hands, shape them into small bite-sized balls and place them back on the parchment paper.
5. Freeze for 1 hour.
Prep Time: 10 minutes

<u>Strawberry Almond Bites:</u>
Ingredients:
-1/2 cup diced strawberries
-1/4 cup almond flakes
-2 tablespoons almond butter
-2 tablespoons honey

Instructions:

1. In a medium bowl, combine diced strawberries, almond flakes, almond butter, and honey.
2. Mix until thoroughly combined.
3. Roll into small balls and place on a parchment-lined baking sheet.
4. Freeze for 1 hour.
Prep Time: 10 minutes

<u>Caramel Coconut Bites:</u>
Ingredients:
-1/4 cup coconut flakes
-1/4 cup almond butter
-2 tablespoons honey
-2 tablespoons caramel sauce
Instructions:
1. In a medium bowl, combine coconut flakes, almond butter, honey, and caramel sauce.
2. Mix until thoroughly combined.
3. Roll into small balls and place on a parchment-lined baking sheet.
4. Freeze for 1 hour.
Prep Time: 10 minutes

<u>Chocolate Cashew Bites:</u>
Ingredients:
-1/4 cup cocoa powder
-1/4 cup raw cashews
-2 tablespoons almond butter
-2 tablespoons honey

Instructions:
1. In a food processor, pulse cocoa powder and cashews until they're combined.
2. Add almond butter and honey and blend until mixed.
3. Line a baking sheet with parchment paper and scoop the mixture onto it.
4. Using your hands, shape them into small bite-sized balls and place them back on the parchment paper.
5. Freeze for 1 hour.
Prep Time: 10 minutes

<u>Peanut Butter Coconut Bites:</u>
Ingredients:
-1/4 cup coconut flakes

-1/4 cup peanut butter
-2 tablespoons honey
-2 tablespoons chia seeds

Instructions:
1. In a medium bowl, combine coconut flakes, peanut butter, honey, and chia seeds.
2. Mix until thoroughly combined.
3. Roll into small balls and place on a parchment-lined baking sheet.
4. Freeze for 1 hour.
Prep Time: 10 minutes

<u>Apple Walnut Bites:</u>
Ingredients:
-1/2 cup diced apples
-1/4 cup walnuts
-2 tablespoons almond butter
-2 tablespoons honey

Instructions:
1. In a medium bowl, combine diced apples, walnuts, almond butter, and honey.
2. Mix until thoroughly combined.

3. Roll into small balls and place on a parchment-lined baking sheet.
4. Freeze for 1 hour.
Prep Time: 10 minutes

<u>Coconut Berry Bites:</u>
Ingredients:
-1/2 cup frozen berries
-1/4 cup coconut flakes
-2 tablespoons almond butter
-2 tablespoons honey

Instructions:
1. In a food processor, pulse frozen berries and coconut flakes until they're combined.
2. Add almond butter and honey and blend until mixed.
3. Line a baking sheet with parchment paper and scoop the mixture onto it.
4. Using your hands, shape them into small bite-sized balls and place them back on the parchment paper.
5. Freeze for 1 hour.
Prep Time: 10 minutes

Coconut Date Bites:
Ingredients:
-1/2 cup coconut flakes
-1/2 cup pitted dates
-2 tablespoons almond butter
-2 tablespoons honey

Instructions:
1. In a food processor, pulse coconut flakes and dates until they're combined.
2. Add almond butter and honey and blend until mixed.
3. Line a baking sheet with parchment paper and scoop the mixture onto it.
4. Using your hands, shape them into small bite-sized balls and place them back on the parchment paper.
5. Freeze for 1 hour.
Prep Time: 10 minutes

Chocolate Berry Bites:
Ingredients:
-1/4 cup cocoa powder

-1/2 cup frozen berries
-2 tablespoons almond butter
-2 tablespoons honey

Instructions:
1. In a food processor, pulse cocoa powder and frozen berries until they're combined.
2. Add almond butter and honey and blend until mixed.
3. Line a baking sheet with parchment paper and scoop the mixture onto it.
4. Using your hands, shape them into small bite-sized balls and place them back on the parchment paper.
5. Freeze for 1 hour.
Prep Time: 10 minutes

 Apple Pie Bites:
Ingredients:
-1/2 cup applesauce
-1/4 cup almond meal
-1 teaspoon cinnamon
-2 tablespoons honey

Instructions:

1. In a medium bowl, combine applesauce, almond meal, cinnamon, and honey.

2. Mix until thoroughly combined.

3. Roll into small balls and place on a parchment-lined baking sheet.

4. Freeze for 1 hour.

Prep Time: 10 minutes

Ingredients:

-2 mashed bananas

-1/4 cup peanut butter

-2 tablespoons honey

-2 tablespoons chia seeds

Instructions:

1. In a medium bowl, combine mashed bananas, peanut butter, honey, and chia seeds.

2. Mix until thoroughly combined.

3. Roll into small balls and place on a parchment-lined baking sheet.

4. Freeze for 1 hour.

Prep Time: 10 minutes

<u>Apple Almond Bites:</u>
Ingredients:
-1/2 cup diced apples
-1/4 cup slivered almonds
-2 tablespoons almond butter
-2 tablespoons honey

Instructions:
1. In a medium bowl, combine diced apples, slivered almonds, almond butter, and honey.
2. Mix until thoroughly combined.
3. Roll into small balls and place on a parchment-lined baking sheet.
4. Freeze for 1 hour.
Prep Time: 10 minutes

<u>Walnut Date Bites:</u>
Ingredients:
-1/2 cup walnuts
-1/2 cup pitted dates
-2 tablespoons almond butter
-2 tablespoons honey

Instructions:

1. In a food processor, pulse walnuts and dates until they're combined.

2. Add almond butter and honey and blend until mixed.

3. Line a baking sheet with parchment paper and scoop the mixture onto it.

4. Using your hands, shape into small bite-sized balls and place them back on the parchment paper.

5. Freeze for 1 hour.

Prep Time: 10 minutes

<u>Peanut Butter Date Bites:</u>

Ingredients:

-1/2 cup pitted dates

-1/4 cup peanut butter

-2 tablespoons honey

-2 tablespoons chia seeds

Instructions:

1. In a food processor, pulse dates and peanut butter until they're combined.

2. Add honey and chia seeds and blend until mixed.

3. Line a baking sheet with parchment paper and scoop the mixture onto it.
4. Using your hands, shape into small bite-sized balls and place them back on the parchment paper.
5. Freeze for 1 hour.
Prep Time: 10 minutes

<u>Chocolate Date Bites:</u>
Ingredients:
-1/4 cup cocoa powder
-1/2 cup pitted dates
-2 tablespoons almond butter
-2 tablespoons honey

Instructions:
1. In a food processor, pulse cocoa powder and dates until they're combined.
2. Add almond butter and honey and blend until mixed.
3. Line a baking sheet with parchment paper and scoop the mixture onto it.

4. Using your hands, shape into small bite-sized balls and place them back on the parchment paper.
5. Freeze for 1 hour.
Prep Time: 10 minutes

<u>Banana Coconut Bites:</u>
Ingredients:
-2 mashed bananas
-1/4 cup coconut flakes
-2 tablespoons almond butter
-2 tablespoons honey

Instructions:
1. In a medium bowl, combine mashed bananas, coconut flakes, almond butter, and honey.
2. Mix until thoroughly combined.
3. Roll into small balls and place on a parchment-lined baking sheet.
4. Freeze for 1 hour.
Prep Time: 10 minutes

<u>Sweet Potato Brownies</u>

Ingredients:
1 cup cooked sweet potato
1/2 cup almond flour
1/4 cup coconut flour
1/4 cup cocoa powder
1/4 cup maple syrup
1/4 cup coconut oil
2 eggs
1 tsp vanilla extract
1/2 tsp baking powder
1/4 tsp salt

Instructions:
Preheat oven to 350°F (175°C).
In a mixing bowl, whisk together sweet potato, almond flour, coconut flour, cocoa powder, maple syrup, coconut oil, eggs, vanilla extract, baking powder, and salt.
Pour the batter into a greased baking dish.
Bake for 25-30 minutes.
Allow to cool before serving.
Prep Time: 10 minutes

Mixed Berry Crumble

Ingredients:
4 cups mixed berries (such as strawberries, blueberries, raspberries, and blackberries)
1/2 cup almond flour
1/2 cup chopped pecans
1/4 cup melted coconut oil
1/4 cup honey
1 tsp cinnamon
pinch of salt

Instructions:
Preheat oven to 375°F (190°C).
In a mixing bowl, combine mixed berries and spread evenly in the bottom of an 8-inch baking dish.
In another mixing bowl, combine almond flour, chopped pecans, melted coconut oil, honey, cinnamon, and salt.
Mix until crumbly and sprinkle over the berries.
Bake for 20-25 minutes or until the crumble is lightly golden brown and the berries are bubbly.

Allow to cool for a few minutes before serving.

<u>Prep Grilled Peaches with Coconut Cream</u>
Ingredients:
4 ripe peaches, halved and pitted
1 can full-fat coconut milk, refrigerated overnight
network error
1 tsp baking soda
1 tsp cinnamon
1/4 tsp nutmeg
pinch of salt
3 eggs
1/4 cup coconut oil, melted
1/4 cup honey
1 cup grated apple (about 1 medium apple)

Instructions:
Preheat oven to 350°F (180°C). Line a muffin tin with paper liners.
In a mixing bowl, whisk together almond flour, baking soda, cinnamon, nutmeg, and salt.

In another mixing bowl, whisk together eggs, melted coconut oil, and honey.
Add grated apple to the wet ingredients and stir to combine.
Gradually add dry ingredients to wet ingredients and mix until just combined.
Spoon batter into prepared muffin tin, filling each cup about 3/4 full.
Bake for 20-25 minutes or until a toothpick inserted into the center of a muffin comes out clean.
Allow muffins to cool before serving.
Prep time: 15 minutestime: 15 minutesCook Time: 30 minutes

<u>Tropical Green Smoothie</u>
Ingredients:
- 1 cup pineapple
- 2 cups spinach
- 1 banana
- 2 tablespoons chia seeds
- 2 cups almond milk

Instructions:
1. Place all ingredients into a blender and blend until smooth.
Preparation Time: 5 minutes

<u>Carrot Cake Smoothie</u>
Ingredients:
- 1 cup carrots, shredded
- ½ cup almond butter
- 2 tablespoons chia seeds
- 1 teaspoon cinnamon
- ½ teaspoon nutmeg
- 2 cups almond milk

Instructions:

1. Place all ingredients into a blender and blend until smooth.
Preparation Time: 5 minutes

Peanut Butter and Jelly Smoothie
Ingredients:
• 2 tablespoons peanut butter
• ½ cup frozen berries
• 1 banana
• 2 tablespoons chia seeds
• 1 teaspoon vanilla extract
• 2 cups almond milk
Instructions:
1. Place all ingredients into a blender and blend until smooth.
Preparation Time: 5 minutes

Tropical Mango Smoothie
Ingredients:
• 1 cup mango
• 2 tablespoons coconut flakes
• 2 tablespoons chia seeds
• 1 teaspoon ginger, freshly grated
• 2 cups almond milk

Instructions:
1. Place all ingredients into a blender and blend until smooth.
Preparation Time: 5 minutes

Blueberry Acai Smoothie
Ingredients:
- 1 cup frozen blueberries
- 2 tablespoons acai powder
- 2 tablespoons chia seeds
- 2 teaspoons honey
- 2 cups almond milk
Instructions:
1. Place all ingredients into a blender and blend until smooth.
Preparation Time: 5 minutes

Green Apple Smoothie
Ingredients:
- 1 green apple, cored and chopped
- 1 banana
- 2 tablespoons chia seeds
- 1 teaspoon ground cinnamon

• 2 cups almond milk
Instructions:
1. Place all ingredients into a blender and blend until smooth.
Preparation Time: 5 minutes

Chocolate Banana Smoothie
Ingredients:
• 1 banana
• 2 tablespoons cacao powder
• 2 tablespoons chia seeds
• 1 teaspoon vanilla extract
• 2 cups almond milk
Instructions:
1. Place all ingredients into a blender and blend until smooth.
Preparation Time: 5 minutes

Strawberry Coconut Smoothie
Ingredients:
• 1 cup frozen strawberries
• 2 tablespoons coconut flakes
• 2 tablespoons chia seeds
• 1 teaspoon vanilla extract

• 2 cups almond milk

Instructions:

1. Place all ingredients into a blender and blend until smooth.

Preparation Time: 5 minutes

Green Protein Smoothie

Ingredients:

• 2 cups spinach
• 2 tablespoons hemp seeds
• 2 tablespoons chia seeds
• 1 teaspoon ground ginger
• 2 cups almond milk

Instructions:

1. Place all ingredients into a blender and blend until smooth.

Preparation Time: 5 minutes

Avocado and Mint Smoothie

Ingredients:

• ½ avocado
• 2 tablespoons fresh mint leaves
• 2 tablespoons chia seeds
• 1 teaspoon honey

• 2 cups almond milk

Instructions:

1. Place all ingredients into a blender and blend until smooth.

Preparation Time: 5 minutes

Pineapple Coconut Smoothie

Ingredients:

• 1 cup pineapple

• 2 tablespoons coconut flakes

• 2 tablespoons chia seeds

• 1 teaspoon ground ginger

• 2 cups almond milk

Instructions:

1. Place all ingredients into a blender and blend until smooth.

Preparation Time: 5 minutes

Matcha Green Tea Smoothie

Ingredients:

• 1 banana

• 2 tablespoons matcha powder

• 2 tablespoons chia seeds

• 2 teaspoons honey

• 2 cups almond milk
Instructions:
1. Place all ingredients into a blender and blend until smooth.
Preparation Time: 5 minutes

Cucumber Mint Smoothie
Ingredients:
• 1 cucumber, peeled and chopped
• 2 tablespoons fresh mint leaves
• 2 tablespoons chia seeds
• 1 teaspoon honey
• 2 cups almond milk
Instructions:
1. Place all ingredients into a blender and blend until smooth.
Preparation Time: 5 minutes

Banana Oat Smoothie
Ingredients:
• 1 banana
• 2 tablespoons oats
• 2 tablespoons chia seeds
• 1 teaspoon ground cinnamon

• 2 cups almond milk
Instructions:
1. Place all ingredients into a blender and blend until smooth.
Preparation Time: 5 minutes

<u>Orange Ginger Smoothie</u>
Ingredients:
• 1 orange, peeled
• 1 teaspoon freshly grated ginger
• 2 tablespoons chia seeds
• 1 teaspoon honey
• 2 cups almond milk
Instructions:
1. Place all ingredients into a blender and blend until smooth.
Preparation Time: 5 minutes

Conclusion

The Whole30 program is a great way to start eating healthier and reset your eating habits. With the help of this cookbook, you can create delicious and nutritious Whole30-compliant meals that will help you stay on track for the duration of the program. Once you complete the 30 days, you should have a better understanding of the foods that work best for your body and the ones that don't. Whether you stick to the Whole30 program or use it as a stepping stone to a healthier lifestyle, you will be on your way to a healthier and happier you! With the recipes in this cookbook, you can create meals that are both delicious and nutritious. Keep in mind that the Whole30 program is not only about the food, but also about creating healthy lifestyle habits. With the help of this cookbook, you can create tasty meals that will help fuel your body and help you stay on track for the duration of the program. Make sure to also take the time to listen to your body and make adjustments when needed. Good luck on your Whole30 journey!

www.ingramcontent.com/pod-product-compliance
Lightning Source LLC
Chambersburg PA
CBHW071100250726
48662CB00019B/1519